SLEEP STRATEGIES

5 STEPS TO SLEEP BETTER AND MASTER YOUR SLEEP HYGIENE

EDWIN GALL

CONTENTS

Intro   v

1. Step One - Environmental Assessment   1
2. Step Two - Schedule Alignment   11
3. Step Three - Tools to Get to Sleep   20
4. Step Four - Ensuring Quality Sleep   34
5. Step Five - Adjusting Sleep-Wake Times   46
6. Putting It All Together   59
7. Resources and Further Reading   68

About the Author   73

INTRO

Welcome to the journey towards better sleep! In the fast-paced world we live in, a good night's sleep is often overlooked, yet it plays a pivotal role in our overall well-being. In this guide, we'll explore the fascinating realm of sleep science and how you can transform your sleeping pattern with 5 steps.

Understanding Sleep Science

Sleep is a complex and essential biological process that impacts every aspect of our lives. From cognitive function to emotional and physical well-being, the quality of our sleep directly influences our daily experiences. By understanding the different sleep states and how they affect our recovery and information processing you'll be better equipped to make informed decisions to improve your sleep. Later in the book, we'll also cover Ultranean sleep cycles as well as sleep Chronotypes that will further your understanding of sleep and assist you in mastering it.

Embracing a Scientific Mindset

No 2 individuals are alike, and the same holds true for our sleep patterns. Different individuals struggle with different sleep problems and so require unique solutions. Recognizing the inherent variability in sleep needs, we recommend adopting a scientific mindset. Think of yourself as a sleep scientist conducting experiments to uncover the optimal sleep solution for you. By approaching the process with curiosity and an open mind, you'll be more receptive to discovering what works best for your unique physiology and challenges.

Common Sleep Challenges

Before we dive into solutions, let's acknowledge the common sleep issues many of us face. Whether it's difficulty falling asleep, staying asleep, or waking up feeling unrested, these challenges are common. Identifying your issues will guide us in tailoring effective strategies to address them. Towards the end of this book, there is a table that provides a comprehensive list of each strategy mentioned throughout the book and whether it assists with falling asleep, staying asleep or waking up in the morning. This should provide a useful guide to help those looking to tailor their approach toward fixing their sleep.

The Power of New Sleep Habits

Research suggests that it takes 18 to 21 days to initiate a new habit and around 66 days for it to become ingrained in your daily routine. Changing your sleep patterns may seem daunting, but understanding the neuroscience of habit change can empower you on this journey.

Consider the brain's remarkable adaptability – as you commit to new sleep habits, your neuronal structures and pathways evolve to accommodate these changes. This neuroplasticity is the key to making your new sleep routine second nature. A quote by motivational speaker Inky Johnson summarises a key point about habit formation and discipline well: "Commitment is staying true to what you said you would do long after the mood that you said it in has left." By embracing discipline and understanding the science behind habit formation, you'll be well on your way to achieving restful nights and energized days.

0.1 The Importance of Quality Sleep

As we begin to better understand our sleep, it's crucial to first understand the profound impact that quality sleep has on our overall well-being. Sleep is not merely a passive state of rest; it is a dynamic and intricate process that contributes significantly to our physical and mental health.

Physical Health and Immune Function

Sleep is a cornerstone of physical health, acting as a powerful regulator of our immune system and hormonal balance. During sleep, the body undergoes essential processes that repair and regenerate tissues, including any damage we've done throughout the day. This includes micro-tears in the muscles throughout the body, leading to muscular growth and strengthening. Additionally, when dieting in a caloric deficit, if you get insufficient sleep your body will atrophy lean muscle mass over fat, as muscle is an active tissue and the body is trying to conserve energy in a sleepless state, making good sleep even more important for body recomposition. Sleep is also when our body regulates and releases many hormones including growth hormone and sex hormones. It is also an important period for our body to focus on fighting off any colds or sicknesses that may be lingering in our bodies. Adequate and quality sleep is integral to maintaining optimal physical health.

Mental Health, Focus, and Productivity

The connection between sleep and mental health is undeniable. Quality sleep enhances our cognitive functions, promoting focus, productivity, and effective decision-making. Additionally, it serves as a natural stress reliever, playing a pivotal role in emotional stabilization. A well-rested mind is better equipped to navigate life's challenges with resilience and clarity.

The Significance of REM Sleep

Rapid Eye Movement (REM) sleep, a phase often associated with vivid dreaming, serves a crucial role in our mental processing. During REM sleep, the brain uncouples connections that are deemed unnecessary, particularly emotions from irrational beliefs. This phase also plays a vital role in forming detailed spatial information, helping us navigate the intricate relationships and rules of our surroundings. The best way to increase the REM sleep you get during the night is to add time to the end of your sleep in the morning, as we get increased REM sleep the longer we are asleep. Avoiding alcohol or THC consumption before bed is also crucial, as these both significantly reduce REM sleep.

The Role of Slow-Wave Sleep

Slow-Wave Sleep (SWS) or Deep Sleep is the phase responsible for motor learning, the consolidation of detailed information, and physical restoration. It acts as a kind of mental filing system, organizing and solidifying memories while supporting the body's recovery from daily wear and tear. Embracing this phase is essential for both mental acuity and physical well-being. To increase Deep Sleep duration, regular timing of sleep is key, as consistency leads to fewer awakenings and deeper sleep.

Exercise during the day is also effective at improving Deep Sleep, as is keeping the ambient temperature in the room cool at night.

Dreams as Processors and Preparers

Dreams, often mysterious and fantastical, play a crucial role in our mental and emotional processing. They are not mere fragments of imagination but serve as tools for preparing and processing situations, including the delicate task of dealing with trauma. REM sleep is also the only time in which our body produces no Adrenaline or Epinephrine, the chemicals responsible for panic and alertness, meaning that we can experience stressful situations in dreams without feeling the stress, helping us to process or prepare for these situations. Understanding the importance of dreams in our sleep cycle adds a layer of appreciation for the intricate ways in which our minds work during the night.

As we unravel the significance of quality sleep, remember that each phase contributes uniquely to our holistic well-being. By recognizing and valuing the diverse roles that sleep plays in our lives, we pave the way for a more intentional and rejuvenating sleep experience.

0.2 The Impact of Poor Sleep

In the hustle and bustle of our daily lives, the repercussions of poor sleep extend far beyond the confines of our bedrooms. The workplace, where we spend a significant portion of our waking hours, often reveals the consequences of inadequate rest. Let's explore the multifaceted impact that poor sleep can have on various aspects of our professional lives.

Waking Times and Tiredness

The morning alarm serves as both a herald and a nemesis for those who've had a restless night. Waking up after insufficient sleep not only disrupts our internal clock but also sets the tone for the day ahead. The restlessness, grogginess and lingering fatigue can cast a shadow over our early hours, affecting our ability to embrace the day with vigor.

Exhaustion and its Ripple Effect

As the day progresses, the exhaustion stemming from poor sleep intensifies. This weariness becomes a pervasive force, infiltrating our tasks and interactions. Simple activities that once felt effortless now lead to a drain on physical and mental reserves. Poor sleep has been shown to lead to increased blood sugar levels, causing greater feelings of tiredness. These blood sugar level increases can be somewhat mitigated by exercising that day, helping to regulate levels again and counterintuitively reducing feelings of tiredness.

Problems Focusing and Productivity

A major impact of poor sleep is the diminished ability to focus and remain productive. Tasks that would typically be approached with precision become daunting challenges. The foggy haze of exhaustion impedes concentration, leading to a frustrating decline in productivity.

Creativity Takes a Hit

Creativity flourishes in well-rested minds. Unfortunately, the lack of quality sleep stifles this creative flow. The vibrant ideas that usually spark innovation and problem-solving become elusive, and the workplace may find itself lacking the dynamic thinking necessary for progress.

Learning Becomes a Struggle

The process of acquiring new skills and knowledge relies heavily on cognitive functions that are compromised in a sleep-deprived state. Poor sleep inhibits the brain's capacity to absorb and retain information, with sleep deprivation significantly inhibiting the ability to retain new memories. This poses a significant obstacle for those seeking professional development or acquiring new competencies.

Social Interactions and People Management

Navigating the intricacies of social interactions and managing people requires finesse and emotional intelligence. Unfortunately, the toll of poor sleep can disrupt these delicate balances. Irritability, mood swings, and a diminished ability to empathize may strain relationships, both with colleagues and those in positions of leadership. Additionally, good sleep has been shown to reduce the perception of others looking angry and increase the perception of others looking happy, having a large impact on how we interact.

The Impact of Poor Sleep on Mental Health

Last but certainly not least, the ramifications of poor sleep extend to mental health. The connection between sleep and mental health is profound and deeply interwoven. In fact, no psychiatric disorder has been identified that maintains a normal relationship with sleep. Poor sleep can severely compromise mental well-being, leading to heightened emotional reactivity, increased susceptibility to anxiety, addiction, and even psychosis.

Emotional Reactivity and Sleep Deprivation

One of the most significant consequences of sleep deprivation is an increase in emotional sensitivity. Research has shown that sleep-deprived individuals experience a 60% increase in amygdala reactivity, the brain region responsible for processing emotions like fear. This heightened reactivity not only makes fearful images appear more threatening, but also causes neutral stimuli to elicit fearful responses. Lack of sleep exaggerates emotional reactions, making it harder to cope with daily stressors and regulate emotions.

REM Sleep and Emotional Processing

Rapid Eye Movement (REM) sleep plays a crucial role in emotional depotentiation, the process by which the emotional intensity of recent memories is diminished. When REM sleep is selectively deprived, as shown in studies, individuals begin to exhibit severe mental health disturbances. By the fifth night, participants displayed psychosis, paranoia, and delusional thinking. Without sufficient REM sleep, the brain struggles to process emotional memories, leading to heightened emotional responses and mental distress.

Impulsivity and Addiction

Sleep deprivation doesn't only amplify negative emotions —it also makes individuals hyper-responsive to positive stimuli. This over-sensitivity can make people more prone to impulsive behaviors and susceptibility to addiction. Moreover, the difficulty in regulating emotions and impulsive behaviors makes it much harder to quit or abstain from addictive substances or behaviors. When individuals are sleep-deprived, maintaining self-control becomes a challenge.

Sleep and Anxiety

Even in individuals with no prior signs of anxiety, sleep deprivation can quickly induce high levels of anxiety.

After just a night of sleep deprivation, over 50% of participants in a study had anxiety levels high enough to qualify for an anxiety disorder. The key contributor here is the lack of deep non-REM sleep. Deep sleep, particularly in non-REM stages, plays a pivotal role in reducing anxiety levels by increasing frontal lobe activity, which is crucial for emotional regulation. This stage of sleep helps shift the body from a fight-or-flight state (sympathetic) to a rest-and-digest state (parasympathetic), lowering cortisol levels, heart rate, and easing the anxiety burden.

Sleep, Suicide, and Nightmares

The link between sleep deprivation and suicidal thoughts is alarmingly strong. Individuals with poor sleep quality are at a higher risk of suicidality, but frequent nightmares are even more predictive of this risk. Nightmares may amplify distress and erode mental resilience, leaving individuals vulnerable to thoughts of self-harm.

Depression and the Importance of Timing

When it comes to depression, the timing of sleep is of utmost importance. Exposure to morning or daytime sunlight, along with the absence of light during the night, has independently been shown to improve mental health outcomes. This reinforces the importance of aligning sleep with the natural light-dark cycle to maintain mental well-being.

Overall, poor sleep not only exacerbates existing mental health conditions but can also be a direct cause of emotional instability, anxiety, and impulsive behavior. Prioritizing deep non-REM and REM sleep, while maintaining consistent sleep timing, is vital for mental and emotional resilience.

Should you happen to have a particularly poor night of sleep when you usually consistently sleep quite well, it is important not to sleep in, go to sleep earlier, nap or consume excess caffeine to offset the poor sleep if you are trying to fix your sleep. This is because it will disrupt your natural rhythm, potentially leading to increased disrupted sleep in the following nights. Aim to go to bed at your usual time and try to resume your routine with as little disruption as possible, with no more than a 30-minute variation in your sleep and waking times. However, if poor sleep is consistent, try to schedule some additional hours of nighttime sleep to make up for the accumulated sleep debt - keeping in mind that it is only possible to catch up on 2 hours of lost sleep per night at best. If you know that later in the week you are going to have a poor night of sleep, such as due to a planned late-night social event, try to get some extra hours of sleep earlier in the week.

In this exploration of the impact of poor sleep on work, it becomes clear that the consequences are not confined to mere tiredness. The workplace, a dynamic arena that demands our best selves, suffers when we neglect the essential foundation of quality sleep. As we journey towards better sleep, we simultaneously pave the way for a more productive, fulfilling, and harmonious professional life.

0.3 The 5 Essential Steps

Embarking on the journey to better sleep involves a strategic and holistic approach. The following 5 steps are the cornerstones of addressing sleep problems, each playing a pivotal role in transforming your sleep experience.

Why the 5 Steps Matter

Understanding the significance of the 5 steps is paramount. These comprehensive measures are designed to tackle sleep issues from multiple angles, providing a holistic and effective strategy for achieving restful nights. By integrating these steps into your routine, you lay the groundwork for sustainable improvements in your sleep quality.

Step 1: Environmental Assessment

Creating an optimal sleep environment is the first crucial step. This includes managing factors like light and temperature to foster a space conducive to rest. In Step 1, look at the intricacies of crafting a sleep-friendly haven to set up a peaceful and undisturbed night's rest.

Step 2: Schedule Alignment

Explore the art of syncing your daily schedule with your body's natural rhythm. Establishing consistent sleep, exercise, and meal schedules forms the backbone of this step. Learn when and why to engage in activities and when to wind down, creating a seamless flow that promotes a harmonious relationship with your body's internal clock.

Step 3: Tools to Get to Sleep

Discover a toolbox of effective techniques to ease into sleep. From body scans to Progressive Muscle Relaxation protocols, explore Non-Sleep Deep Rest methods and harness the power of an auditory toolkit. These tools act as allies in calming the mind and paving the way for a tranquil transition into restful sleep.

Step 4: Ensuring Quality Sleep

Quality sleep goes beyond just getting to bed; it involves strategic planning and mindful choices. This step empowers you to make informed decisions that enhance your overall sleep experience. Uncover the influence of pre-bed activities, dietary considerations, and caffeine consumption on the quality of your sleep.

Step 5: Adjusting Sleep-Wake Times

Understand the rhythm of your Circadian clock and learn strategies to synchronize your sleep cycle with it. Explore techniques for adjusting sleep-wake times and discover the art of strategic napping to boost daytime performance. This step allows you to fine-tune your sleep patterns for optimal efficiency.

The key to success lies in the collective implementation of each of the 5 Steps. Together, these steps form a comprehensive guide that addresses the nuanced aspects of sleep, offering you a pathway to nights filled with restorative and rejuvenating sleep.

Before We Begin

This book offers practical insights into non-pharmacological sleep strategies primarily to suggest potential methods backed by scientific inquiry that may positively influence your sleep. It is not intended to delve into intricate scientific details, but provides further reading suggestions for those seeking a deeper understanding. While these strategies may enhance sleep quality for many, this book is not tailored to address chronic diagnosable sleep conditions. Individuals with serious persistent sleep concerns are strongly advised to seek the guidance of qualified professionals.

It is crucial to consult with your medical professional or clinician before implementing any strategies outlined in this book, especially if you have pre-existing health concerns. The influence of medications and supplements on sleep is not covered here, and readers are encouraged to consult specialists for personalized recommendations. While this book focuses on non-pharmacological approaches, it does not replace professional advice, and any potential supplements or medications should be discussed with a healthcare professional.

Readers are advised to follow the recommended approach of reading each chapter in consecutive order and implementing changes gradually. Trying to make all adjustments simultaneously may prove challenging to maintain. This book emphasizes a holistic, step-by-step process for achieving better sleep, and promoting long-term well-being.

ONE

STEP ONE - ENVIRONMENTAL ASSESSMENT

Welcome to the first crucial step on your journey to transforming your sleep: the Environmental Assessment. Your sleep environment is not merely a backdrop for your nightly adventures in dreamland; it's a powerful determinant of the quality of your rest. Below we will cover the profound impact of creating a sleep-friendly space and delve into the nuances of managing light and temperature to lay the foundation for a restful night.

In the realm of sleep improvement, your environment is your ally. By the end of this chapter, you'll be equipped with the knowledge and tools to curate a sleep sanctuary that invites tranquillity and supports your journey to better sleep. Let's dive into the first step – your Environmental Assessment – and unlock the secrets to transforming your bedroom into a haven for restorative sleep.

1.1 Creating a Sleep-Friendly Environment

The space in which you rest should be viewed as more than just a room; it's a sanctuary for rejuvenation. Let's explore the key elements to curate a sleep-friendly space that promotes restful nights and sets the stage for the first step on your sleep-improvement journey.

The surroundings in which you lay your head profoundly influence the ease with which you drift into a peaceful slumber and how well you stay asleep. We'll uncover the importance of crafting a space that embraces restfulness, free from distractions and disruptions.

Ensure Proper Ventilation Throughout the Night

Fresh air is not just invigorating; it's a vital component of a conducive sleep environment. Ensure proper ventilation in your bedroom to optimize air circulation throughout the night. A well-ventilated room contributes to a comfortable and restorative sleep experience. This will assist in improving air quality, humidity and temperature. You may either choose to ventilate by keeping a door or window open, depending on the weather and living circumstances. Air conditioning is another option, however, be aware that this may lead to very dry air which may affect sleep quality.

Dedicate Your Bed to Sleep and Intimacy

The bed is a sacred space for sleep and intimacy. By refraining from using it for other activities, you condition your brain to associate the bed exclusively with rest. Aim for more than 90% of your time in bed to be dedicated to sleeping, reinforcing the bed as a sanctuary for peaceful slumber. Using the bed for other activities, such as watching TV or using your phone for entertainment may lead your brain to associate the room with entertainment rather than sleep, making it more difficult to slip into a calm and restful state.

Embrace Dim Lighting for Evening Serenity

As the night unfolds, transition into a serene atmosphere by introducing dim lighting below eye level. Soft, ambient lighting signals to your body that it's time to wind down, paving the way for a smoother transition into sleep. Bright overhead lights will imitate daytime sunlight and lead to greater levels of alertness and wakefulness, particularly as the light gets directly into your eyes from overhead. Overhead light and light below eye level is the key distinction, as the angle of the light matters for reprogramming our Circadian Rhythm. Our eyes interpret artificial light as if it were sunlight, so overhead light is interpreted as midday sun - a key time for alertness and productivity - whereas light below eye level imitates sunrise or sunset.

Therefore, it is key to avoid direct light exposure close to bedtime by using lighting below eye level and dimming the lights as much as possible. Where possible and safe to do so, candles or fireplaces are ideal as the level of light they produce will not lead to further wakefulness.

Blockout Curtains for Darkness and Privacy

Unwanted light, whether from street lamps or the moon, can disrupt your sleep cycle. Blockout curtains serve as a shield against unnatural light, creating a dark and private cocoon that enhances your body's melatonin production and fosters an ideal sleep environment. This can also be helpful during months when the sun rises before you wish to wake. Ideally, you want curtains that can still be drawn first thing in the morning, as this immediate sun exposure will help the waking process.

Banish Electronic Devices from the Bedroom

Resist the temptation to bring devices like televisions, computers, or smartphones into your sleep sanctuary. The blue light emitted from screens interferes with your circadian rhythm, disrupting the natural signals for sleep. Additionally, these devices are designed to be engaging and stimulating, hence using these late at night will be counter-productive to sleep. Create a tech-free zone that encourages relaxation and unwinding. If possible, even charge your phone outside the room, as using it within an hour of trying to sleep will be disruptive. Removing the temptation will be the most effective way to avoid this.

Ditch the Clockfaces for Stress Reduction

Clock-watching induces unnecessary stress and anxiety about the passing of time. Remove clockfaces from your bedroom to eliminate the temptation to check the hours throughout the night. By letting go of the clock, you free your mind from the pressure and allow a more natural flow into a restful sleep. This can also apply to those who track their 'sleep scores' too closely and experience anxiety around a poor score. A study showed that participants who were lied to about their sleep score performed better in a physical event when they thought they slept better. If sleep score anxiety is an issue, it may be effective to only check it once a week or take a break from tracking for a while.

Elevate Feet for Glymphatic Support

Enhance the glymphatic washout process by elevating your feet while sleeping. This simple adjustment supports the efficient removal of toxins from the body, promoting deeper sleep and aiding in recovery. Some sources suggest that sleeping on your side can also assist with glymphatic washout. Elevating your feet or sleeping on your side may become a subtle yet impactful technique for optimizing sleep depth.

By implementing the strategies above, you'll be creating a sleep sanctuary that beckons you to rest and rejuvenate. As we delve further into the intricacies of creating a sleep-friendly environment, remember that small changes can yield significant improvements in the quality of your sleep.

1.2 Managing Light Exposure

Mastering the art of managing light exposure is essential for setting the stage for a restful night's sleep. Let's unravel the nuances of light exposure and discover how sunlight can be harnessed to orchestrate our circadian rhythm for better sleep.

Sunlight: A Morning Elixir

The first rays of morning sunlight herald more than the dawn; they set the stage for a day of vitality and well-being. Here's your guide to embracing the early sun and unlocking a cascade of benefits for your body and mind.

Aim to expose yourself to direct sunlight within the initial 30 to 60 minutes of waking if you want to shift your Circadian Rhythm. Ensure that if this isn't possible your morning sunlight exposure occurs before approximately 10 am, as from around 10 am till 3 pm is known as the "Circadian Dead Zone", where direct sunlight will not have an effect on shifting your Circadian Rhythm.

Aim for sunlight exposure between 10 minutes on sunny days to 20 minutes on cloudy days, as this acts as a potent catalyst for setting your Circadian Rhythm. Ideally, this sunlight should be received outside - through a normal window or from under partial cover can be less effective substitutes if weather is an issue. Be cautious of viewing the sun through other barriers such as a car window, as the tinting will block out the necessary light to have the desired effects. Where the sun is not visible at all, bright overhead lights can have a similar effect, though not nearly as potent.

While basking in the morning glow, remember to never stare directly into the sun. Such an action is not only unpleasant but can be harmful to your eyes. Simply being outside will result in enough sunlight directly into your eyes to garner the desired positive effects.

The efficacy of this morning ritual lies in the intensity of light it delivers. Aim for an exposure that equates to about 100,000 LUX, a unit measuring light intensity. This optimal luminance triggers a series of physiological responses, setting your Circadian Rhythm to initiate the waking process around that time in the morning. As mentioned above, you will get approximately 100,000 LUX from 10 minutes of direct sunlight exposure outdoors on a sunny day and 20 minutes on an overcast day. Sunlight through a window (particularly tinted windows) will provide significantly less LUX.

This early sunlight exposure becomes a cue for your body to release cortisol, a hormone that plays a pivotal role in jumpstarting your day. Cortisol isn't just an awakening agent; its presence in the morning positively influences your immune system, metabolism, and focus throughout the day.

The benefits extend beyond the physiological. Revel in the mood enhancement, increased energy levels, and regulated appetite that this morning sunlight imparts. Moreover, dopamine release is boosted, contributing to a sense of well-being and motivation.

In summary, aim for between 10 to 20 minutes of direct sunlight exposure each morning before 10am to reset your Circadian Rhythm to the rising and setting of the sun. Incorporate this simple yet powerful practice into your morning routine. Whether the sun emerges in all its brilliance or peeks behind clouds, let the morning light be your ally. As you immerse yourself in this daily ritual, you'll find your days infused with vitality, focus, and a sense of well-being.

Sunset: Nature's Lullaby

As the day wanes, welcome another dose of direct sunlight around sunset. This afternoon exposure acts as a gentle signal for bedtime, aiding those who struggle with sleep onset or waking up. Additionally, it counterbalances the effects of late-night screens, mitigating their impact on your sleep-wake cycle. This will help shift your Circadian Rhythm closer to the sunset viewed, particularly helpful if you struggle to get to sleep at night or wake in the morning. Remember, do not stare directly into the sun, simply being outside will result in the amount and angle of sunlight exposure to receive the positive benefits of the sunset.

Blue Light Banishment

In the hours leading up to sleep, create a sanctuary of dim lights, candles, or fireplace glow. Steer clear of blue light emanating from electronics at least an hour before bedtime. The magic of these dim lights is not just in their soothing ambiance but in their ability to preserve dopamine levels, warding off feelings of depression and anxiety. Protect your sleep environment from bright overhead lights an hour before bedtime to maintain this delicate balance.

Eye Masks

In unfamiliar sleep environments or amidst disruptive light, consider the use of eye masks. These tools act as guardians of your sleep, regulating external stimuli and creating a cocoon of tranquillity.

As we navigate the delicate balance of light, remember that these elements are not merely external factors but integral components affecting your sleep biology. By controlling their influence, you take a significant stride toward harmonizing your sleep patterns and embracing restful nights.

1.3 Temperature Control: Embracing Your Internal Thermal Clock

The Goldilocks principle (or the "just right" principle) applies not only to porridge and planets but also to the temperature of your sleep space. We'll unravel the science behind finding the "just right" temperature for optimal rest. Discover how to create a cool and comfortable sleep haven, optimizing your body's natural cooling process for a restorative night's sleep.

Morning Wake-Up Call: Cold Showers and Ice Baths

Kickstart your day with an invigorating crescendo by incorporating cold showers or ice baths in the early hours. If these aren't possible, cold water on the face, hands and feet can also provide some benefit. Beyond the bracing wake-up effect, these chilly rituals stimulate the nervous system and promote alertness. They act as a refreshing prelude to a day of vitality, setting the tone for heightened wakefulness. The cold shock will trigger the release of a neurotransmitter known as norepinephrine, leading to greater levels of alertness and focus.

Additionally, it will cause your body to cool down, leading your body's natural regulatory mechanisms to heat you back up, counterintuitively leading to an increased core body temperature. This heating process results in your average body temperature rising, which is conducive to a 'waking' Circadian Rhythm, meaning you will feel more awake and alert long after the initial shock of the cold wears off.

As well as the benefits to wakefulness and alertness, cold showers and ice baths also have benefits for fat loss and reducing the stress response - shivering in the cold will lead to greater fat loss whereas resisting shivering will lead to a greater tolerance to stress. Please implement this strategy with caution, as it is advised you consult with a healthcare professional before jumping straight into a cold shower or ice bath if you have any pre-existing health conditions. There is no need to shower for a long period of time in the cold to achieve these benefits. Working up to a 2-minute cold shower should provide the vast majority of the benefits from the cold.

Evening Serenade: Warm Showers for Temperature Regulation

As the day winds down, a warm shower or bath is not only an effective way to relax but also to prepare for sleep. If a shower or bath isn't possible, submerging hands, face and feet in warm water can provide some benefit as well. Contrary to the morning ritual, a hot shower in the evening again serves a counterintuitive purpose—cooling down the body. This thermal shift in the body's internal temperature regulation after a shower creates a conducive environment for the onset of restful sleep. After the initial rise in body temperature from the hot water, your body will begin cooling itself down again after you get out. This cooling process lasts long after you dry off. The cooling of your body signals your Circadian Rhythm that it is time to sleep and also leads to deeper sleep at night. Notably, aging also leads to poorer thermal regulation, leading to potential insomnia. As hot baths cause vasodilation, this can improve thermal regulation, making this strategy even more effective in older individuals.

Bedroom Bliss: Cool Environment and Adjustable Blankets

Maintain a cooler environment in the bedroom, as research suggests that a drop in body temperature is directly related to both falling asleep and quality of sleep. Equip your bed with blankets that are easily removable, ensuring adaptability to your body's changing temperature needs during the night. Studies indicate the ideal cool ambient temperature is around 65.3°F (18.5°C). This simple yet effective strategy allows you to cocoon yourself in comfort and facilitate deeper sleep.

Visualize the ebb and flow of each element of temperature control working together to build a harmonious atmosphere for restful sleep. From the invigorating chill of morning cold showers to the comforting warmth of evening routines, every component synchronizes to establish an ideal thermal setting for rejuvenation. With temperature as a supportive companion, allow the nighttime ambiance to lead you into a state of revitalizing slumber.

TWO

STEP TWO - SCHEDULE ALIGNMENT

Welcome to the core of your sleep journey – Step 2: Schedule Alignment. In the steady flow of life, consistency takes the lead, and timing is the guiding force. In this chapter, we'll explore the significance of syncing your schedule, from the early hours of the morning to the serene moments preceding sleep. We'll also explore 1 of the core frameworks for good sleep - the QQRT acronym by sleep expert Dr Matthew Walker. Let's examine the timing that shapes the tranquil rhythm of restful nights.

2.1 Establishing a Consistent Sleep Schedule: The QQRT Approach

In the complex tapestry of sleep, consistency is the golden thread that weaves together the fabric of restful nights. Establishing a consistent sleep schedule is essential to improving sleep quality, regulating appetite, and enhancing overall well-being. Let's break down the key components of a consistent sleep schedule using the QQRT framework: Quality, Quantity, Regularity, and Timing.

Quality: Measuring the Effectiveness of Your Sleep

The quality of your sleep is as important as the number of hours you spend in bed. Quality can be assessed by measuring the percentage of time you are actually asleep versus the total time you spend in bed. High-quality sleep is essential for effective rest, recovery, and cognitive function. Consistently maintaining a high sleep quality fosters the kind of rest that allows your body to rejuvenate and your mind to sharpen. A consistent sleep schedule enhances this quality by training your body to recognize when it's time to rest, optimizing your deep sleep and slow-wave sleep stages.

Quantity: Ensuring Sufficient Sleep Hours

Quantity refers to the total number of hours you spend asleep each night. Adequate sleep quantity is crucial for maintaining optimal physical and mental health. Research indicates that sleep plays a vital role in regulating hunger-related hormones like leptin and ghrelin, which influence appetite control. A consistent sleep schedule helps ensure that you get enough sleep each night, allowing your body to replenish energy stores, cleanse the build-up of adenosine—a chemical that causes sleepiness—and wake up feeling refreshed. No other animals in the animal kingdom artificially wake themselves up, so if you often wake up still feeling tired or find yourself needing more sleep, it may indicate sleep deprivation.

Regularity: Synchronizing Your Sleep-Wake Patterns

Regularity is the consistency with which you go to sleep and wake up at the same time each day. Minimizing the difference in your sleep and wake times to no more than 30 minutes, even on weekends, helps synchronize your body's internal clock. This synchronization supports the natural release of sleep-inducing melatonin in the evening and cortisol in the morning, optimizing both sleep onset and wakefulness. A study showed that students who slept the same number of hours each night at the same time performed better in cognitive tests than those who slept more hours but inconsistently at various times, indicating that regularity also increases the quality of sleep. Consistently sleeping at the same times each day fosters the kind of quality sleep that nourishes your body and mind, as your body learns when it is time to rest and recover. Regularity is a linchpin for achieving adequate deep sleep and slow-wave sleep, the essential stages that contribute to physical rejuvenation and cognitive function.

Timing: Aligning Sleep with Your Chronotype

Timing refers to the specific hours of the day you sleep and wake, matched against your chronotype—whether you are naturally a morning person or a night owl. We will explore Chronotypes in more depth in a later chapter, but for now it is enough to understand the importance of sleeping to your natural rhythms. Aligning your sleep schedule with your natural biological rhythms enhances the restorative effects of sleep. Additionally, understanding your Ultradian Sleep Cycles—approximately 90-minute cycles of light and deep sleep—can help you wake up at an optimal time, avoiding grogginess. By setting your sleep duration in approximate multiples of 90 minutes (e.g., 6 hours, 7.5 hours, or 9 hours), you can ensure that you wake up at the end of a sleep cycle, feeling more alert and refreshed. Remember however that these cycles are not exactly 90 minutes long for everyone, so do not stick to them too closely, or you may end up interrupting a cycle instead of naturally waking at the end of a cycle.

Establishing a consistent sleep schedule through the QQRT approach (focusing on Quality, Quantity, Regularity, and Timing) will guide you toward better sleep and overall well-being. By paying attention to these aspects, you'll be well on your way to harnessing the full restorative power of sleep.

2.2 When Should You Exercise and Eat?

In the coordination of sleep optimization, the timing of your exercise and meals has the influence to organize a sequence of energy, focus, and rest. Let's delve into the strategic practice of aligning physical activity and nutrition with the inherent flow of your day and night.

Morning Cardio: Wake Up the Body and Mind

Rise with the sun and kickstart your day with cardiovascular exercise. This morning ritual not only trains your body to wake up but also acts as a powerful catalyst for focus and alertness throughout the day. Engaging in regular cardiovascular exercise such as running, bike riding, swimming or even a brisk walk at the same time each morning will condition your body to release the waking hormone cortisol before you open your eyes to wake you for the anticipated exercise. The invigorating effects of morning cardio will set a vibrant tone for the hours ahead.

Daytime Resistance Training: Energize for the Day, Sleep Better at Night

Beyond its immediate wake-up call, resistance exercise offers a unique bonus for nighttime slumber – an increase in slow-wave sleep. Resistance training can include lifting free weights, using exercise machines, resistance bands and bodyweight exercises. Training with resistance will lead to microtears in the muscles that will then repair as you sleep. This repair process leads to a deeper state of sleep at night. However, steer clear of intense training sessions within 2-3 hours of bedtime to avoid disrupting your ability to fall asleep and disrupting the depth of your sleep.

Timing Your Meals: Eating to Your Internal Clock

When you eat your meals plays a pivotal role in shaping both your waking and sleeping times. Eating earlier in the day can adjust your waking time, while evening meals can nudge your body towards a later bedtime. Recognize the influence of timing your meals on your body's internal clock and use it to your advantage.

Intermittent Fasting: Morning Focus Boost

Embrace intermittent fasting, particularly in the critical morning period. By delaying your first meal until midday, you prevent your body from expending energy on digestion, channeling more blood to your brain for enhanced focus and productivity. This strategic approach to eating supports your morning routine and primes you for a day of heightened mental acuity.

Meal Size and Composition: Lunch as the Culmination

Timing when you eat larger portions of your daily food can have significant effects on the quality of sleep, energy levels, alertness and getting to sleep. Breakfast is often known as the "Most important meal of the day" and it is often where people tend to go wrong. If you feel you cannot skip breakfast altogether, having a small carbohydrate-free breakfast instead will provide similar effects, avoiding the typical tiredness that often accompanies a 'carb coma'. When looking to be focused, productive and alert, avoiding a carbohydrate-rich breakfast is key - stick primarily to fats and protein first thing in the morning.

Having lunch as the largest meal of the day (where you consume most of your calories) during the early hours of the afternoon ensures that your body has ample time to digest and convert food into usable energy.

If you're seeking a gentle nudge towards sleep, consider incorporating complex low-gi (i.e. avoiding sugar) carbohydrates around 2 hours before bedtime to both facilitate a sense of tiredness and fill your muscles with energetic glycogen for the morning when you wake for the day. A bit of self-experimentation may be necessary to find the right time to stop eating before bedtime, but data suggests eating within 1 hour of bedtime is disruptive to sleep.

Hydration Wisdom: Balance for Restful Nights

Be mindful of your water intake, especially close to bedtime. Excessive water consumption before sleep can diminish the amount of REM sleep you experience. This is particularly important if your sleep is often disturbed by the need to use the bathroom throughout the night. Strike a balance that keeps you adequately hydrated while preserving the integrity of your nighttime rest. Attempting to drink the majority of your water by 3 pm can help you to reach your hydration goals without suffering the negative effects on sleep. If this method does not suit you, attempt to have your last large drink 3 hours before bedtime, with only small sips (such as to take medications) within 3 hours of going to bed. Do not attempt to sleep within 20-30 minutes of swallowing any tablets as lying flat will impede your ability to digest tablets and may lead to indigestion.

In this subsection, we've navigated the intricate intersections of exercise and nutrition, uncovering the strategic timing that enhances both your waking hours and your nights of restful slumber. As you fine-tune your daily routine, the timing of your exercise and meals become allies that increase your vitality and rejuvenation.

2.3 Creating Waking and Wind-Down Schedules

The moments right after waking and just before bedtime set the cadence for your day and night. Let's explore the art of tuning waking and wind-down schedules into rituals that harmonize with your body's natural rhythms.

Consistent Morning Routine: A Decision-Making Sanctuary

Imagine your morning routine as a sanctuary of decisions already made. By establishing consistency through a regular routine, you conserve precious decision-making energy for the challenges that lie ahead, avoiding crashing into decision fatigue early in the day. This is especially crucial if you often find yourself grappling with morning grogginess. Create a structured routine that guides you seamlessly into the day, minimizing the mental clutter of choice.

Morning Sunlight Exposure: A Wake-Up Elixir

As the day unfolds, invite the sun into your waking hours. Exposure to sunlight for 10-20 minutes each morning serves as a natural cue, setting your Circadian Rhythm in motion. Open curtains wide to welcome the light, kickstarting your body's alertness. Consider incorporating light walking, stretching, or cardiovascular exercise to further awaken your body and mind while getting your morning sunlight.

Scheduled Morning Joy: A Motivational Boost

Knowing there's something enjoyable waiting for you can be a powerful motivator, adding a touch of excitement to your wake-up ritual. Infuse your morning routine with a preferred activity, a delightful rendezvous that beckons you out of bed. Whether it's savoring a cup of coffee, engaging in a hobby, or simply relishing a quiet moment, let anticipation be the catalyst that propels you into the day. Feeling a sense of achievement can also help to create a sense of momentum throughout the day, so planning something productive first thing can also be effective.

Consistent Nighttime Routine: The Prelude to Rest

As the day winds down, transition into a consistent nighttime routine. Signal to your body that it's time to unwind and prepare for sleep. Embrace the slight boost of alertness that often precedes bedtime due to a release of hormones, using this time to engage in and complete your nighttime rituals.

Screen-Free Sanctuary: Dimming the Lights for Sleep

About an hour before bedtime, create a screen-free sanctuary. Dim overhead lights and avoid screens to allow your body to naturally wind down. Ideally, charge your phone outside the bedroom, relying on an alternate alarm to awaken you. This not only reduces screen time but also minimizes potential sleep disruptions from notifications.

Example Morning Routine:

• 6:30 AM: Open curtains for initial morning sunlight

• 6:45 AM: Light stretching or a short walk in the sun

• 7:00 AM: Engage in a preferred morning activity

• 7:30 AM: Prepare a nutritious breakfast

• 8:00 AM: Begin the work or daily activities with a clear and focused mind

Example Nighttime Routine:

• 8:30 PM: Dim overhead lights, switch to ambient lighting

• 8:45 PM: Charge phone outside the bedroom

• 9:15 PM: Complete a brief mindfulness or relaxation exercise

• 9:30 PM: Engage in a calming activity (reading, gentle stretching)

• 10:00 PM: Set the alarm clock, tuck into bed for a restful night

By creating waking and wind-down schedules that align with your natural rhythms, you transform transitions into rituals and routines that guide you seamlessly into restful nights and vibrant mornings.

THREE

STEP THREE - TOOLS TO GET TO SLEEP

In this chapter, we explore the tools designed to guide you gently into the embrace of sleep. Step 3 unveils an array of tools—from body scans to auditory aids—that redirect the mind, calm the nervous system, and pave the way for a tranquil night's rest. If you often struggle with an overactive mind at night, the key to getting to sleep is to do whatever you can to get your mind off itself and stop excessive rumination. The tools provided in this chapter are various methods to assist with this goal.

These tools not only redirect the mind but also play a pivotal role in calming the parasympathetic nervous system (PNS). For those who grapple with nightmares as a result of trauma, these tools can be a soothing, calming, gentle road to healing and respite.

3.1 Body Scans and PMR Protocols

In the realm of sleep assistance, Body Scans and Progressive Muscle Relaxation (PMR) protocols offer a gateway to relaxation, calming the nervous system, and guiding the mind and body into a state conducive to restful sleep. Let's unravel the essence of Body Scans and PMR, providing you with practical steps to start on your journey into the land of dreams.

What is a Body Scan?

A Body Scan is a mindfulness practice that involves directing focused attention to each part of your body. This intentional awareness, like a gentle spotlight, moves systematically from head to toe or vice versa. The purpose is to release tension, promote relaxation, and redirect your focus away from the buzzing thoughts that may hinder your ability to sleep.

How does it help with sleep?

A Body Scan serves as a bridge from the external world to the internal sanctuary of your body. By relaxing into the sensations in each individual part of your body, you cultivate a sense of calm and presence. This deliberate shift from the chaos of the day and all the thoughts buzzing around inside your head to the tranquillity within prepares your mind and body for the serenity of sleep.

Example Body Scan Script:

Step 1: Settling In

Close your eyes gently and take a few slow, deep breaths. Inhale relaxation, exhale tension. Allow each breath to carry you deeper into a state of calmness.

Step 2: Focusing on Breath

Shift your awareness to your breath. Feel the gentle rise and fall of your chest and abdomen with each inhalation and exhalation. Breathe naturally, letting go of any need to control your breath.

Step 3: Starting with the Toes

Bring your attention to your toes. As you inhale, notice any sensations within each toe—tingling, warmth, or the subtle weight against the surface. Exhale, allowing the sensations to unfold. Take 3 slow, deep breaths, focusing on the sensations.

Step 4: Moving to the Feet

Shift your focus to the soles of your feet. Inhale and sense the points of contact with the bed. Exhale, feeling any subtle sensations in your feet. Take 3 slow, deep breaths, immersing yourself in the sensations.

Step 5: Journeying Up the Legs

Progress upward, scanning your awareness through your ankles, calves, and knees. Inhale slowly and feel the weight of your legs against the bed and the points of contact between the surface and your legs. Take 3 slow, deep breaths, focusing on any sensations in your legs.

Step 6: Hips and Pelvis

Bring your attention to your hips and pelvis. Inhale deeply, sensing the subtle movements in this area. Exhale, feeling any sensations. Take 3 slow, deep breaths, immersing yourself in the sensations.

Step 7: Abdomen and Lower Back

Shift your awareness to your abdomen and lower back. Inhale calmly, feeling the expansion of your belly. Exhale, sensing any subtle movements. Take 3 slow, deep breaths, focusing on the sensations.

Step 8: Chest and Upper Back

Continue to your chest and upper back. Inhale deeply, feeling the rise and fall of your chest. Exhale, savoring any sensations in this area. Take 3 slow, deep breaths, immersing yourself in the sensations.

Step 9: Shoulders

Direct your attention to your shoulders. Inhale, lifting them slightly. Exhale, feeling any tension dissolve. Take 3 slow, deep breaths, focusing on the sensations in your shoulders.

Step 10: Arms and Hands

Shift your focus to your upper arms, forearms, and hands. Inhale, sensing any warmth or weight in your arms. Exhale, feeling the sensations unfolding. Take 3 slow, deep breaths, immersing yourself in the sensations.

Step 11: Relaxing the Neck

Bring your awareness to your neck. Inhale deeply, sensing any movements or warmth. Exhale, feeling the subtle release of tension. Take 3 slow, deep breaths, focusing on the sensations in your neck.

Step 12: Jaw and Face

Now, shift your attention to your jaw and face. Inhale, sensing any sensations in your facial muscles. Exhale, allowing the jaw to relax. Take 3 slow, deep breaths, immersing yourself in the sensations.

Step 13: Slow Full-Body Scan

Inhale deeply as you slowly scan from the bottom to the top of your body. Exhale, feeling the sensations along the way. Slowly move your attention from the tips of your toes to the top of your head over the course of 3 deep, slow breaths, focusing on any sensations you feel along the way.

Step 14: Full-Body Integration

Feel the accumulated sensations from your toes to the top of your head. Inhale deeply, savoring the sensation of calmness. Exhale slowly, focusing on the sensations throughout your body. Try to fill your whole body with awareness at once and sense your body as a whole.

What is PMR?

Progressive Muscle Relaxation is a technique that involves tensing and then relaxing different muscle groups in sequence. By intentionally creating tension and then releasing it, PMR promotes a profound state of physical and mental relaxation. It serves as a gentle conductor, guiding your body into a tranquil repose.

How does it help with sleep?

PMR is akin to a gentle massage for the entire body, unraveling the knots of tension accumulated throughout the day. By systematically relaxing each muscle group, PMR not only calms the nervous system but also creates physical and mental relaxation, paving the way for restful sleep.

Example PMR Script:

Step 1: Getting Comfortable

Close your eyes gently and take a few slow, deep breaths. Inhale through your nose, hold for a moment, and exhale through your mouth. Release any overall tension you may be holding in your body from the day.

Step 2: Focusing on Your Breath

Shift your attention to your breath. Feel the natural rhythm of your breathing. Inhale relaxation, exhale tension. Allow each breath to bring you a sense of calmness.

Step 3: Progressive Muscle Relaxation

We'll now systematically tense and then release each muscle group, starting at the head and working down to the feet. As you tense each muscle, hold for a few seconds, and then release the muscle on the exhalation, focusing on the sensation of relaxation.

Face:

○ Scrunch your facial muscles, creating tension in your forehead, cheeks, and jaw.

○ Hold for a moment.

○ Release on the exhalation, letting go of any facial tension. Feel your face becoming smooth and calm.

Neck:

○ Gently tilt your head back, tensing the muscles in your neck.

○ Hold briefly.

○ Release on the exhale, allowing your neck to return to a comfortable position. Feel the ease in your neck.

Shoulders:

○ Lift your shoulders towards your ears, creating tension.

○ Hold for a few seconds.

o Release on the exhale, letting your shoulders drop down. Feel the stress melting away.

Chest:

o Take a deep breath, expanding your chest.

o Hold for a moment.

o Release on the exhale, releasing any tightness in your chest.

Biceps:

o Tighten your biceps by bringing your arms close to your body.

o Hold briefly.

o Release on the exhale, experiencing the release of tension.

Forearms:

o Flex your forearms, tightening the muscles.

o Hold briefly.

o Release on the exhale, allowing the muscles to soften. Feel the gentle flow of relaxation.

Hands:

o Clench your fists tightly, feeling the tension.

o Hold for a few seconds.

o Release on the exhale, letting go of all tension. Feel the warmth and relaxation in your hands.

Stomach:

o Tighten your abdominal muscles.

○ Hold briefly.

○ Release on the exhale, letting go of any residual tension.

Thighs:

○ Tense the muscles in your thighs by pressing your legs together.

○ Hold for a few seconds.

○ Release on the exhale, feeling the muscles loosen.

Calves:

○ Point your toes towards your body, creating tension in your calves.

○ Hold for a moment.

○ Release on the exhale, allowing your calves to relax completely.

Step 4: Full Body Relaxation

Take a moment to scan your body. Feel the overall sense of relaxation spreading from the top of your head to the tips of your toes. Enjoy the soothing sensation of calmness and tranquillity.

3.2 Non-Sleep Deep Rest (NSDR) Practices: A Sanctuary for the Mind

In the realm of sleep optimization, Non-Sleep Deep Rest (NSDR) practices emerge as versatile tools, offering a variety of benefits beyond the pursuit of sleep. This section unveils the magic of NSDR, shedding light on its ability to calm the nervous system, quiet the mind, and provide profound rest even when sleep remains elusive. Let's explore the diverse landscape of NSDR, from meditation to hypnosis, and discover the tranquillity each practice offers.

What are NSDR Practices?

Non-Sleep Deep Rest practices encompass a variety of techniques designed to induce a state of deep restfulness without necessarily leading to sleep. These practices create a sanctuary for the mind, calming the nervous system and ushering you into a serene space of tranquillity.

How do they assist with sleep?

Non-Sleep Deep Rest (NSDR) practices serve as conduits between wakefulness and sleep, adeptly guiding the mind and body into a state of repose. By soothing the nervous system, they lay the groundwork for a seamless transition into the serene realm of sleep. Beyond their potential to induce sleep, these practices confer a multitude of benefits. They aid in memory retention, fostering improved cognitive functions and enhancing rates of neuroplasticity, thereby promoting optimal learning.

As stress melts away under the influence of NSDR, individuals may experience not only relief but also a heightened ability to manage pain. The restorative nature of these practices also contributes to enhanced sleep quality, while simultaneously sharpening focus and mental clarity. In essence, NSDR practices not only prepare the path to sleep but also offer a haven for the mind, nurturing various facets of well-being when full sleep cannot be achieved.

NAPS: A MINIATURE RETREAT

Napping is an NSDR practice, offering a brief yet effective respite for the mind. Keeping it short (15-20 minutes) can avoid entering deep sleep and potentially disrupting your nighttime slumber and feelings of grogginess.

MEDITATION: CULTIVATING STILLNESS

Meditation is a timeless NSDR technique, guiding you into a state of deep rest by focusing the mind and calming the nervous system. Apps like Headspace or Insight Timer can be valuable companions on your meditation journey, providing guided meditations and other tools to facilitate a meditative state.

HYPNOSIS: A GUIDED RESPITE

This NSDR practice involves inducing a state of heightened suggestibility, allowing your mind to enter a deep restful state. The link at the end of this book to Reveri provides access to scripts supported by scientific research.

YOGA NIDRA: YOGIC SLEEP

Yoga Nidra, or yogic sleep, is a profound NSDR practice that combines deep relaxation with guided meditation to enter a sleep-like state for deep rest when sleep cannot be reached. Explore the links at the end of this book to yoga nidra scripts on YouTube for an immersive experience in deep rest.

These NSDR practices, endorsed by Neuroscientist Dr. Huberman through his podcast Huberman Lab, beckon you into a realm of tranquillity. Whether you choose the gentle embrace of a nap, the mindful stillness of meditation, the guided journey of hypnosis, or the yogic sleep of Yoga Nidra, NSDR practices become the pillars supporting your nightly quest for rejuvenation and repose.

3.3 Auditory Sleep Toolkit: A Symphony of Serenity

This section unveils the magic of auditory tools, exploring how these melodic companions can assist in the journey to sleep and deeper, more rejuvenating slumber. Enlist the support of auditory tools to create a harmonious sleep environment. Whether it's soothing nature sounds, background noise or calming music, auditory aids redirect your focus away from external distractions.

How can Auditory Tools Assist with Sleep?

Auditory tools are like lullabies for the mind, creating a soothing ambiance that aids in relaxation and guides the mind away from the hustle and bustle of the day. Not only do they assist in washing out any disturbing noises in and around your house, but they can also help to override the engaging thoughts that sometimes keep us awake. Some evidence even suggests that particular background sounds can induce brain waves more conducive to restful sleep. Auditory tools can serve to coax your mind into a tranquil state where sleep becomes a natural progression.

It is worth noting that while there are many upsides, there are also potential drawbacks to these tools. Becoming reliant on a particular noise playing to get to sleep can become limiting if used too often, leaving you sleepless on nights when the sound is unavailable. In addition, some evidence suggests that having background noise playing can take some brain space as the mind works to block it out of conscious awareness while sleeping, leading to a less deep state of rest (although other evidence suggests that particular frequencies lead to a deeper state of rest). Considering this, it is recommended that these auditory tools be used as an aid to sleep when sleep is difficult to capture, rather than a routine tool to use every night.

Diverse Auditory Tools: Your Personalised Sleep Soundscape

NATURE SOUNDS:

Immerse yourself in the natural sounds of Earth like rain, ocean waves, falling water, woods, or wilderness. These sounds mimic the calming rhythms of nature, transporting your mind to tranquil landscapes and facilitating a peaceful transition to sleep.

COLOR NOISES:

Embrace the spectrum of color noises, each with its unique frequency profile, including white noise, pink noise and brown noise. White noise, resembling static, can mask background sounds, while brown and pink noise offers deeper, more natural tonalities that promote relaxation. While there is a degree of preference in which to listen to, at the time this book was written there was more evidence for pink noise than white noise for improving sleep.

BINAURAL BEATS:

Experience the dance of frequencies with binaural beats. By presenting slightly different tones to each ear, binaural beats create a perceived third tone, encouraging brainwave synchronization, and increasing Alpha brain waves, which are associated with a relaxed and restful state of mind. Different frequencies can induce states of relaxation, aiding in the journey to sleep.

BEDTIME STORIES:

Rediscover the comfort of bedtime stories. Whether read or narrated, these tales provide a gentle distraction for the mind, easing it into a state of restful repose. It is best to listen to a story that you have heard before and to avoid listening to any content that teaches new things, as anything too engaging will discourage sleep as your mind will be active and stimulated.

ASMR RECORDINGS:

ASMR (Autonomous Sensory Meridian Response) recordings are designed to evoke tingling sensations and a sense of calm. From whispers to tapping sounds, ASMR can be a delightful addition to your auditory sleep toolkit.

RELAXING MUSIC WITH LOW BPM:

Melodies with a gentle rhythm and soothing tones can create a peaceful atmosphere, inviting your mind to unwind. Music with a low BPM (Beats Per Minute), anything from around 60-80 BPM is ideal. Also, consider music without lyrics to prevent excess mental stimulation.

Creating Your Personalised Soundscape

Experiment with different auditory tools to discover what resonates with your senses. Whether it's the rhythmic patter of rain, the gentle hum of white noise, or the melodic embrace of soothing music, curate a personalized sleep symphony that guides you effortlessly into the tranquil realm of restful slumber. As you embark on this auditory journey, let the melodies become the companions that lead you into the serenity of sleep.

3.4 Taking a Mental Walk

Our final strategy to assist with falling asleep is the mental walk. This simple strategy has shown surprising effectiveness for those who struggle to sleep at night. Simply close your eyes and try to vividly envision yourself walking a route you are very familiar with and find relaxing. This could be around your local neighborhood, somewhere in nature or to your local cafe. Imagine the walk in as much detail as possible, picturing the sights, smells and sounds that are familiar to you. Take your time and do not rush the walk, try to really imbed yourself into the experience and relax into it. Many find themselves softly drifting off to sleep before they ever reach their destination.

Note: try not to become too reliant

While the sleep tools above can assist in inducing sleep or encourage a deeper slumber, remember to be cautious of becoming too reliant on these tools to achieve sleep. The ultimate goal should be to reliably achieve sleep without the need for these tools, however, they are available in times when sleep is elusive.

FOUR

STEP FOUR - ENSURING QUALITY SLEEP

Welcome to a pivotal stage of your sleep journey, where we look into the essence of quality sleep. Step 4 goes beyond the conventional notion of time in bed, unraveling the intricate nature of sleep duration and, more importantly, sleep quality. In this chapter, we explore the profound impact of not just how long you sleep but the depth and restorative nature of that sleep. Let's explore why it's not merely about the hours spent in bed but the rejuvenation hidden within those nocturnal hours.

The Importance of Sleep Duration: More Than Meets the Eye

We often measure our sleep success by the hours we spend in bed. However, your mere presence in bed does not equate to the restorative slumber our bodies and minds crave. Quality sleep is not solely a numbers game; it's about the profound impact those hours have on your overall well-being.

Decoding the Equation: Duration vs. Quality

Consider this: 8 hours in bed does not guarantee 8 hours of blissful, restorative sleep. The quality of your sleep—the depth of your journey into the various sleep stages—is equally, if not more, crucial. It's about the efficiency of your sleep, the way your body and mind move through the cycles of rejuvenation.

What Defines Sleep Quality?

Quality sleep is characterized by the harmonious progression through sleep stages, from the initial drowsiness of Non-REM (Non-Rapid Eye Movement) sleep to the vivid dreams of REM (Rapid Eye Movement) sleep. It involves the orchestrated release of hormones, cellular repair, and the rejuvenation of both mind and body.

Why Does Sleep Quality Matter?

The benefits of quality sleep extend far beyond feeling rested in the morning. It influences cognitive function, emotional well-being, immune strength, and even metabolic health. In essence, it's not just about the duration, but the efficiency of the restorative process that occurs during those precious hours of slumber.

4.1 Strategic Activity Planning Before Bed: Unwinding the Mind

The moments leading up to bedtime set the stage for the quality and duration of the restoration throughout the night. To ensure both duration and quality, strategic activity planning before bedtime becomes essential. This involves winding down activities, avoiding stimulants like caffeine (including any food or drinks that contain caffeine, like some teas and soft drinks), and creating a conducive environment that signals to your body that it's time to transition into the restorative phases of sleep.

The Power of Less Engaging Activities

As the night descends, the mind craves activities that gently coax it into a state of relaxation. Engaging in less stimulating pursuits becomes the key to quality sleep. This is not the best time for intellectual acrobatics or learning new skills, exploring new ideas or understanding new concepts but rather a time to enjoy a gentle descent.

Reading: A Literary Lullaby

When approached with a mindful selection, reading becomes a literary lullaby for the mind. Choose materials that are not intellectually challenging or stimulating, as these may get your mind racing when you mean to drift off peacefully to sleep. Let the words flow gently, creating a bridge between the bustling activities of the day and the serenity of sleep. A mere 10 to 20 minutes can work wonders in easing the mind into a calm state. General examples may include informative non-fiction factual books (the kind you are mildly interested in rather than fascinated by), relaxing fiction or non-fiction books, and books that you have read before work great as well. Try to avoid anything that is too contemplative, suspenseful, emotionally gripping, or thought-provoking.

The Device Dilemma: An Hour of Respite

In the final hour before sleep, bid farewell to your digital companions. Devices emit stimulating blue light that interferes with the natural circadian rhythm, signaling to your brain that it's time to be alert. Additionally, these devices and the apps they contain are designed to capture your attention and keep your mind stimulated so you continue to use them. Decades of research have gone into the neuroscience of attention and how the reward pathways in the brain (utilizing Serotonin, Dopamine, etc.)

lead to prolonged attention. Social media companies in particular utilise this research in the design of their applications to hold your attention hostage for as long as possible, as longer engagement with their applications means more profits for the company as you engage with more advertisements. Embrace an hour of respite, allowing your mind to disengage from the digital world and gradually transition into a state of restfulness.

Defer Serious Discussions: A Nocturnal Pact

Serious or heavy discussions, akin to caffeine for the mind, are best deferred to the daytime. Engaging in weighty conversations just before bed stirs the mental waters, making it challenging for the mind to settle into the serene depths of sleep. These stressful conversations can often lead to releases of Adrenaline/Norepinephrine and cortisol, leading to feeling wired and an increased sense of wakefulness and alertness. Save these discussions for a time when the mind is rested and alert.

Create a Soothing Ritual

As you navigate the delicate balance of winding down, consider crafting a pre-sleep ritual that speaks to your senses. Whether it's the warmth of herbal (not caffeinated) tea, a relaxing stretching routine, a warm shower, or the gentle rustle of pages turning, let your ritual become a soothing melody that signals to your mind that it's time to surrender to the embrace of sleep. Refer back to subchapter 2.3 Creating Waking and Wind-Down Schedules where we discussed this further.

4.2 The Influence of Diet on Sleep

In the culinary balance of life, what you consume not only fuels your waking hours but plays a vital role in your resting hours. Below we unravel the delicate influence of diet on sleep—where timing, choices, and awareness become the characteristics that determine the quality and depth of your nightly rest.

From the timing of meals to the impact of caffeine, understanding the relationship between diet and sleep is a crucial aspect of crafting an environment conducive to both sleep duration and quality.

Making Sleep-Friendly Culinary Choices: The 1-Hour Rule:

To allow your body to shift its focus from digestion to repair, it's wise to avoid eating within 1 hour of bedtime and avoid heavy meals within at least 2 hours before bed. The digestive process requires a significant amount of energy and blood flow to facilitate, meaning these resources are redirected away from other important restorative tasks during sleep. Lying horizontally also interferes with the digestive process, particularly when your stomach is very full, and can lead to indigestion which may prevent you from falling asleep. By adhering to the 1-Hour Rule, you ensure your body isn't occupied with the demands of digestion while trying to sleep.

Cultivating Sleep-Friendly Eating Habits: The Ritual of Mindful Eating

Approach your evening meal mindfully. Select nourishing, sleep-friendly options that won't burden your digestive ensemble. Whole foods, lean proteins, and complex carbohydrates should make up the final meal of the day, supporting your body's readiness for rest. Consuming a meal before bed consisting of more complex carbohydrates may induce a greater feeling of drowsiness (a 'Carb coma'). Avoid any foods high in sugar as the blood glucose spike will increase energy levels and alertness. Just remember the 1-hour rule and avoid eating within 1 hour of trying to sleep as a later mealtime may push back your Circadian Rhythm and lead to you sleeping and waking later.

Hydration

While sipping on water is encouraged throughout the day, be mindful of excessive fluid intake just before bedtime. This ensures that you won't be interrupted by midnight calls to the bathroom, allowing your body to remain in the restful rhythm of sleep. Excessive fluid consumption right before bedtime has been associated with reduced REM sleep. It's recommended that you consume most of your water for the day before 3 pm to avoid frequent nighttime trips to the bathroom.

Alcohol: The Deceptive Sedative

While a nighttime alcoholic beverage may seem like a tempting prelude to slumber, alcohol is a deceptive sedative. It may initially induce drowsiness, but as you drift off to sleep, it disrupts the delicate sequencing of sleep cycles, the depth of sleep, and the pattern of sleep. It will punctuate your sleep with frequent waking that you do not remember and significantly disrupt your REM sleep. Understanding alcohol's influence on sleep is essential for making conscious decisions about when to consume it.

Marijuana

The shadows of marijuana can obscure the clarity of your sleep, ushering you into initial drowsiness. However, its impact on the natural sleep architecture can result in fragmented slumber and diminished sleep quality, interference with dreams, and disruption of the sleep cycles and depth of rest.

Regular marijuana users often report a cessation of dreams during sleep. This is due to the REM sleep-disrupting quality of THC, 1 of the primary active chemicals in Marijuana. When users cease consuming Marijuana, there is often a 'REM sleep rebound' where dreaming temporarily becomes more intense to make up for the deficit.

The other active primary chemical in Marijuana is CBD. This reportedly has less negative effects on sleep, though research is still being conducted. However, CBD is known to often have an anxiolytic (anxiety-reducing) effect and can reduce core body temperature, which may act as a direct sleep-improving mechanism.

Relying on marijuana to induce sleep may pose a risk of sleeplessness if access is limited, hindering the development of essential sleep skills and neglecting to address other contributing factors leading to poor or elusive sleep. Consistent use can also lead to tolerance, requiring higher doses to achieve the same results. There is additionally often withdrawal-induced insomnia when many users cease consuming after consistently using Marijuana to sleep long term.

Sleep Medications

Certain sleep medications may also cast shadows on the clarity of your sleep, inducing initial drowsiness but affecting the natural sleep architecture. Dependence on sleep medications may heighten the risk of sleeplessness without access or upon awakening during the night. This reliance could also thwart the development of essential sleep skills and neglect addressing broader environmental, psychological, or physiological factors contributing to elusive sleep. Melatonin may also fall into this category, as regularly consuming this hormone can disrupt the natural production of Melatonin in the body as well as other hormones related to quality sleep. Nevertheless, there is a place for sleep medications in specific circumstances, and guidance from healthcare professionals, such as doctors and psychiatrists, should be sought.

Other Drugs

Be mindful of the influence of other drugs on your sleep. Some medications, whether prescription or over-the-counter, may have unexpected effects on your nightly rest (for example, many medications contain caffeine). This can include antidepressants such as SSRIs (Selective Serotonin Reuptake Inhibitors), which have been known to induce Insomnia in many cases, which may be considered counterproductive as a known common symptom of Insomnia is depression. Consulting with a healthcare professional about potential sleep disruptions is crucial for informed choices.

4.3 Caffeine Consumption and Timing: Mastering the Elixir of Alertness

In today's fast-paced world, caffeine often plays a key role in keeping us energized and focused. It's a widely enjoyed stimulant that can enhance alertness, but it's important to consider its effects on sleep. By understanding how caffeine interacts with our bodies, especially when it comes to timing and moderation, we can enjoy its benefits without compromising our rest. Below, we explore how to balance caffeine consumption with maintaining healthy sleep habits.

How does Caffeine work?

The primary mechanism of caffeine is that the caffeine molecule blocks the Adenosine receptors in the brain, as caffeine attaches to the receptors because it has a similar molecular structure. Adenosine is known to induce tiredness so this is why caffeine makes you feel awake, as it stops Adenosine from binding to the Adenosine receptors - the process that makes you feel tired.

However, in addition to this mechanism, caffeine also activates noradrenaline neurons and affects the local release of dopamine and interactions with serotonin, thought to also induce wakefulness. Both your metabolism of caffeine (how quickly your body processes it) as well as your sensitivity to caffeine (how much of an effect a dose of caffeine has on your body) are important when considering caffeine consumption.

How Caffeine Affects Sleep: Balancing Benefits with Sleep-Friendly Practices

Caffeine can be a helpful stimulant that enhances alertness and focus, but its timing and amount are key to preserving good sleep quality. By blocking adenosine, a chemical that accumulates in the brain and promotes sleepiness, caffeine keeps you alert, but it can also interfere with the natural sleep cycle. When caffeine is still active in your system close to bedtime, it may cause difficulties falling asleep, more frequent waking, and a reduction in slow-wave sleep, which is crucial for feeling refreshed.

The 8-Hour Rule: Timing Caffeine to Support Sleep

To maintain restful sleep, it's recommended to avoid caffeine at least 8 hours before bedtime. For some people, caffeine can remain active even longer, some research indicating up to 14 hours, so finding your own cut-off time through experimentation is helpful. Larger doses in the morning and tapering off as the day progresses can be an effective strategy to enjoy caffeine's benefits while ensuring it doesn't interfere with your night's rest.

The Morning Grace Period: Delay Early Caffeine Intake

Although many of us reach for caffeine as soon as we wake up, waiting 90 minutes after waking before consuming caffeine can better align with the body's natural rhythm. In the morning, your body releases cortisol, which helps you wake up naturally. Drinking caffeine immediately can disrupt this process, leading to an energy dip later in the day. By waiting, you can help your body wake up naturally and maintain stable energy throughout the day.

Finding the Balance: The 400 mg Limit

Both the FDA and sleep expert Dr. Matthew Walker recommend keeping daily caffeine intake within 400 mg, the equivalent of about three to four cups of coffee. This moderate amount allows you to enjoy the benefits of caffeine, such as improved focus and mood, without increasing the risk of sleep disturbances or dependence. It is worth noting that this is a generalized recommendation, as the optimal daily intake will be influenced by a variety of factors, including age, size, and tolerance. However, generally staying within this limit will assist regular consumers to optimize the benefits while avoiding potential negative consequences.

Consider Periodic Abstinence for Resensitization

Regular caffeine consumption leads to tolerance, requiring higher and higher doses to achieve the same feelings or alertness while increasing the metabolic burden on the body. Regular use of caffeine can also change the neurobiology in your brain, leading to increased feelings of tiredness when caffeine is not in the system. With regular caffeine use the brain becomes used to having the Adenosine receptors blocked, so when caffeine isn't present we feel even more tired. If you find caffeine tolerance or dependence continues to increase, consider an abstinence period of 2-4 weeks a few times per year to allow your brain to resensitize to the presence of caffeine.

Long-Term Health and Caffeine

In moderate amounts, caffeine has been shown to improve concentration and performance, particularly under conditions of sleep deprivation. However, some research indicates that consistent overconsumption may delay the brain's recovery from adenosine build-up, which can affect cognitive functions related to memory and learning. Moderation helps prevent long-term disruption to brain health, while allowing you to enjoy caffeine's positive effects.

Caffeine and Daytime Performance

Caffeine can boost alertness and performance, especially when you're tired, but it's important to note that it often restores performance diminished by fatigue rather than enhancing it beyond normal levels. Consistent daily caffeine use can also be associated with sleep disruptions, leading to a cycle where poor sleep necessitates more caffeine, potentially impacting daytime energy levels. By being mindful of your intake and timing, you can benefit from caffeine without negatively affecting your sleep quality.

By respecting the recommended 400 mg daily limit and timing your caffeine consumption thoughtfully, you can maximize its benefits while safeguarding both your sleep and overall health.

Tailoring Caffeine to Your Circadian Rhythm

Aligning caffeine intake with the natural peaks and troughs of your energy levels, you can take full advantage of the effects of this stimulant. Consider when your energy levels and focus usually plummet throughout the day and when you need to be alert and focused, and time your caffeine for these key periods. Caffeine reaches peak plasma levels and hence effectiveness around 17-20 minutes after consumption, so consider this when timing your caffeine throughout the day.

Experimenting with Timing: Finding Your Optimal Caffeine Cadence

As you aim to master caffeine consumption and timing, allow room for experimentation. Everyone's sensitivity to caffeine is unique, and by fine-tuning the timing, you can uncover the cadence that resonates with your body's own sleep and wake cycles.

By understanding the delicate balance of timing and moderation, you transform caffeine into a supportive partner in the flow of daily life, allowing you to savor both the vigor of alertness and the tranquillity of rest.

FIVE

STEP FIVE - ADJUSTING SLEEP-WAKE TIMES

Welcome to the final act of your transformative journey toward better sleep. Step 5 beckons us into the realm of adjusting sleep-wake times. Consider this step not merely as a finale but as a prelude to a new chapter— where your sleep aligns seamlessly with the cadence of your aspirations and vitality.

Common Challenges in Sleeping and Waking

Before diving into the next section, it's important to address some common challenges that may affect your ability to get to sleep or wake up. Ensure you consider the following when trying to adjust your sleep-wake times.

1. Investigate the potential influence of sleep disorders or other mental health diagnoses

Sleep disorders lurk in the shadows, often undetected. From insomnia to sleep apnea, these conditions demand attention. Seeking professional guidance for diagnosis and treatment is a pivotal step. Additionally, the influence of stress and anxiety can turn our minds into a whirlwind, making it challenging to relax and initiate sleep. Seeking

Cognitive Behavioural Therapy (CBT) to specifically address sleep issues has been shown to have some success in reducing Insomnia. Prioritizing mental health, adopting relaxation techniques, and seeking the appropriate support are paramount.

2. Plan sufficient wind-down time at night

The modern pace of life can leave us rushing into bedtime without properly winding down. Failing to allocate time for relaxation before sleep can disrupt the transition from wakefulness to rest. It is also a common problem to sit down after a long and busy day, only to realize it is almost the time when you want to sleep, but you haven't had any time to relax or engage in activities of your choosing. This can lead to engaging in these activities at the expense of your sleep. Make sure to prioritize this time for yourself at night. End or postpone tasks that are not urgent to give yourself sufficient wind-down time to engage in activities of your choosing.

3. Prioritise consistency

This is particularly important in your bedtime, waking times, duration of sleep as well as your daily routine (regular exercise and mealtimes will help with sleeping). As mentioned throughout the book, consistency is key to conditioning your Circadian Rhythm, as each part of your daily routine acts as an 'indicator' to your internal clock as to whether it is time to be alert and awake or winding down for sleep. Ensure your bedtime and waking times are the same each day (as close as possible - within 30 minutes daily) and the number of hours you sleep is consistent. Ensure your daily exercise happens around the same time each day, as your body will release natural hormones to prepare you for the bout of physical exertion. Similarly, your body will also wake up or wind down to when it expects the first and last meals of your day.

Consequences of Poor Sleep

Embarking on a journey towards better sleep is not just about the pursuit of nightly rest; it's about steering clear of the pitfalls that come with sleep deprivation. Poor sleep jeopardizes not only our energy levels but also our cognitive prowess.

Picture a foggy morning where focus falters, creativity wanes, and productivity takes a nosedive. Beyond the mental effects of sleep deprivation, the physical toll is significant, with weakened immunity and a heightened vulnerability to health issues. Additionally, mood swings also result from a lack of adequate sleep. Given the combined deficits in mental clarity, physical health, and mood stability, the pursuit of good sleep is a journey worth taking, for in the realm of rest lies the power to rejuvenate both mind and body. Remember, the goal is improvement, not perfection.

Understanding the 80/20 Rule

You don't need to nail your sleep-wake schedule every night to witness transformative changes, just as you do not need to implement every single strategy in this book to master your sleep. By achieving the desired sleep rhythm 80% of the time, you pave the way for substantial improvements in sleep quality and overall well-being.

Freedom in Imperfection

Allow imperfection to be your ally on this journey. Life is dynamic and ever-changing, and your sleep-wake times can ebb and flow. Grant yourself the freedom of imperfection on your sleep journey, knowing that each step towards improvement is a victory in itself.

Envision the challenges of adjusting sleep-wake times not as obstacles but as opportunities for growth. It is important to remember that, like watching the clock tick from your bed as you try to sleep, fixating on perfection will likely lead to more harm than good. As you embrace the 80/20 rule, embrace imperfection, and prepare to transform your sleep.

5.1   Finding   Your   Circadian   Rhythm   and Chronotype

Adjusting your sleep-wake times requires a deep dive into the intricate mechanisms of your body's internal clock. In this section, we unravel the enigma of your Circadian Rhythm and Chronotypes—2 pillars that shape the cadence of your waking and slumber.

The Circadian Rhythm Unveiled

The Circadian Rhythm is a natural, internal process that regulates the sleep-wake cycle, repeating roughly every 24 hours. It regulates sensations of alertness, tiredness, body temperature, and even appetite and thirst throughout the day via periodic releases of hormones and neurotransmitters. The Circadian Rhythm primarily tracks the time of day via light exposure, with heat exposure as a secondary measure. It operates to coordinate biological processes to occur consistently at the best times each day to maximize performance for the individual. Understanding its nuances is key to guiding your body through the movements of the day.

As mentioned above, along with light exposure, temperature also plays a key role in your Circadian Rhythm. Your body temperature fluctuates alongside your Circadian Rhythm throughout the day (these fluctuations are small, around 97.7–99.5°F (36.5–37.5°C) with the coolest point being about 2 hours before you wake (your Temperature Minimum) and the warmest point being about 2 hours before you sleep (your Temperature Maximum).

While measuring this is somewhat impractical (you would need to measure your average hourly resting core body temperature), knowing when your body is in a 'warming' or 'cooling' state can be useful for adjusting your Circadian Rhythm.

Your body will typically be in a 'warming' state from when it reaches your temperature minimum (about 2 hours before you usually wake) till it reaches your temperature maximum (about 2 hours before you usually sleep). A warming state indicates you are in the waking cycle of your Circadian Rhythm. During this time, More light exposure will amplify the waking signal, as well as cold water immersion to raise your core body temperature (while counter-intuitive, homeostatic processes in your body will work to raise your core body temperature in response to the cold water).

Your body will then enter a 'cooling' state when it reaches your temperature maximum (about 2 hours before you usually sleep) till it reaches your temperature minimum (about 2 hours before you usually wake). This cooling state indicates you are in the wind-down/sleeping cycle of your Circadian Rhythm. During this time, reduced light exposure and warm water immersion will assist the wind-down cycle.

Chronotype Demystified

A Sleep Chronotype is your individualized sleep preference —a unique cycle that dictates whether you're an 'early bird' or a 'night owl'. Understanding your Chronotype sheds light on the optimal times for wakefulness and rest.

Discovering Your Chronotype

While no rigid categories define Chronotypes, a continuum stretches from early risers to late-night sleepers. To discover your place on this spectrum, explore the nuances of your preferences and habits. Are you naturally alert in the morning or do your energy levels peak in the evening? If you don't already have a good idea of what your chronotype is, you can take a free quiz to discover where your tendencies lie. To delve deeper into your Chronotype, take the free quiz at: https://qxmd.com/calculate/calculator_829/morningness-eveningness-questionnaire-meq

Age, Genetics, and Chronotypes: Unravelling the Threads

Age and genetics play a part in determining your Chronotype, yet they don't dictate the entire story. Typically, up to the age of 20, more people tend towards early rising. From 20 to 30 individuals tend more towards a night owl chronotype, then from 30 onwards the chance of being an early riser progressively increases with age. However, environmental, psychological, and physiological cues hold sway, offering opportunities for adaptation and transformation.

In this exploration of Circadian Rhythm and Sleep Chronotypes, deciphering the rhythms of your internal clock and understanding your Chronotype provides insight into the optimal times for wakefulness and rest and also unlocks the potential to harmonize your sleep-wake times with the natural cadence of your life.

5.2 Strategies to Adjust Your Sleep Cycle

Embarking on the quest to align your sleep-wake times requires a strategic approach—a series of nuanced steps that delicately guide your body's internal clock. In this section, we lay out some practical strategies to adjust your sleep cycle, offering a roadmap to synchronize your slumber with the cadence of your aspirations. 3 strategies are outlined in this section: Sleeping Backward; Sleep Scheduling and Sleeping Forward. These strategies are outlined in order of how drastic they are, with Sleeping Backward having minimum impact on your daily life and Sleeping Forward having the largest impact, due to how it will affect your daytime routines during implementation. As only 1 of these 3 strategies can be used at a time, it is recommended that if more than 1 strategy is attempted, they are tried in this order.

1. Sleeping Backward

For those seeking a more measured approach, consider sleeping backward. Counterintuitive to the end goal, it is best to start by moving bedtime forward one hour to ensure you are tired and ready for sleep, then make subtle adjustments of 15-30 minutes each night until your sleep aligns with your desired schedule. This meticulous approach allows you to finely tune your sleep-wake times without overwhelming your body's internal rhythm.

For example, if you usually sleep at 12 am but want to sleep at 10 pm, you would initially set your bedtime at 1 am the first night; then 12:30 am the second night; 12:00 am the third night; and so on until you reach 10 pm.

2. *Sleep Scheduling*

This strategy focuses on initially limiting your total time in bed so you spend more time in bed sleeping and less time trying to get to sleep. Remember that more than 90% of the time you spend in bed should be spent sleeping if you want to sleep effectively.

Set your bedtime when you expect rapid sleep onset to occur soon after you lie down. Ensure to then set an alarm that is the average number of hours you usually spend asleep after your bedtime. For example, you usually fall asleep at 1 am after lying in bed for 2 hours and sleep for about 4.5 hours. On your first night of Sleep Scheduling you would then set your bedtime at 1 am and set an alarm to wake up at 5:30 am)

As sleep efficiency improves and you are sleeping consistently between your set bedtime and waking time, incrementally increase your total time in bed by 15-minute intervals each night. Adjust the time in bed to match your desired sleep schedule. Using the example above, once you are sleeping consistently between your sleep-wake times and you want to bring your bedtime earlier, set your bedtime for 12:45 am the next night instead of 1 am.

Continue to increase this interval by another 15 minutes only when you are consistently falling asleep at the newly set bedtime.

This approach increases total sleep while finely tuning your sleep-wake times. This approach is best for those who struggle to fall asleep soon after they initially get into bed or who struggle to increase their time asleep.

3. Sleeping Forward 2 Hours Each Night

When sleeping forward, imagine your sleep adjustment as a gradual march towards your desired sleep time. In this strategy, you progressively shift your bedtime forward by 2 hours each night until you arrive at your target. For example, if you usually sleep at 12 am and want to sleep at 10 pm, the first night you would go to bed at 2 am; the second night at 4 am; the third night at 6 am; and so on until you reach 10 pm.

This incremental approach allows your body to acclimate gradually, minimizing resistance and facilitating a smoother transition. This strategy is most effective for those who struggle to bring back their bedtime and sleep earlier in the night but have no problem staying up later. You will of course also need a flexible schedule to accommodate during the transition, as your bedtime will be changing dramatically each night, so this will not work while also trying to attend a normal 9-5 job.

Key Points to Remember When Adjusting Your Sleep Cycle

Whichever strategy you choose to apply from the 3 outlined above, it is also important to remember the impact time in bed, napping and sunlight exposure can have upon resetting your sleeping time.

Time in Bed

In the quest for rest, it is common to spend hours in bed, struggling to get to sleep and lying there in frustration. This often just leads to more sleeplessness as you become increasingly worried you will not sleep. To counteract this, set a specific window to attempt falling asleep. If after lying there for this time slumber still eludes you, take a brief intermission. Get up, engage in a relaxing activity in dim light, such as stretching, listening to a podcast or reading a book, and return to bed only when drowsiness beckons. Strictly avoid eating, bright lights or looking at screens during this time, as this will wake you further. Dr Matthew Walker recommends not to lie in bed trying to sleep for more than approximately 20-25 minutes.

This strategy proves particularly effective in addressing difficulties settling in bed for sleep and inappropriate sleep timing. Even accounting for the break from attempting to sleep, those who struggle with sleep will usually end up sleeping faster using this strategy than if they simply lay there in frustration.

Appropriate Napping

While the allure of daytime sleep may be tempting, it poses a challenge in adjusting your sleep cycle. If daytime napping is unavoidable, keep it brief—set an alarm for 20 minutes—to avoid disrupting nighttime slumber. More information on napping strategically will be covered in the next section.

Sunlight Exposure

As mentioned previously, viewing sunlight as close to sunrise and sunset as possible will signal your Circadian Rhythm to reset to daylight hours. With many of us living primarily indoor lifestyles, it is surprisingly easy to miss this critical light exposure, so our Circadian Rhythms often become dysregulated. Make sure you get your light exposure at these critical times of day if you are serious about rectifying your sleep schedule.

By embracing these nuanced approaches, you not only guide your body towards harmonious sleep-wake times but also cultivate effective habits that resonate with the rhythms of your vibrant, waking life.

5.3 Strategic Napping for Performance: Unleashing the Power of Midday Rejuvenation

Strategic napping can be a powerful tool for assisting feeling rested, improving performance and revitalization. In this section, we explore the art and science behind napping, revealing how brief moments of repose can elevate your performance and enhance your waking life.

The Benefits of Strategic Napping

Napping is more than a momentary escape, it's a strategic act of rejuvenation. A well-timed nap serves as a miniature reset button for your mind and body. Naps can offer a reset to your emotional state, a slight upward mood boost, enhanced alertness, and a revitalized cognitive capacity. A short nap will help reduce the build-up of adenosine in your brain, reducing feelings of tiredness and providing a boost to alertness and concentration.

If you often struggle to fall asleep for a nap, some quick tips include taking off shoes, blocking out light, reducing noise, and using a blanket. Don't forget to set a timer!

Nap Duration and Timing for Optimal Performance

Nap duration and timing hold the key to maximizing benefits without falling into the pitfalls of sleep inertia - that feeling of grogginess, disorientation, drowsiness, and cognitive impairment that can often come straight after waking up. Managing your nap duration can help you to acquire the desired benefits from your nap, rather than falling asleep and hoping for the best.

A nap duration between 45-90 minutes will provide you with a comprehensive refresh, allowing your body to run through a full sleep cycle, however, this will very likely lead to sleep inertia, or grogginess, after waking.

If you desire a boost to alertness, brain energy, focus, and motivation while avoiding that groggy feeling from your nap, the sweet spot remains between 15-20 minutes, which allows you to reap the rewards of a nap without entering the deeper stages of sleep that may lead to grogginess upon waking. Less than 15 minutes and the benefits are little and not sustained, and any more than 20 minutes exponentially increases the chances of experiencing sleep inertia.

Nap to Improve Learning

Optimize your learning by taking a post or mid-learning nap. Napping after a study session or intense learning bout has been shown to enhance memory consolidation, improving the retention of new information. It also improves the connection and integration of new knowledge, helping to make more associations, ideas, and solutions with the newly learned information. Napping midway through a learning bout has also been shown to have benefits, increasing learning of the study session by 20% after the nap, as well as being able to sustain longer learning sessions.

Nap in the Afternoon or After Lunch

During the day, our levels of alertness vary according to our Circadian Rhythm. We are usually more alert in the morning, then in the early to mid-afternoon we experience a 'postprandial dip', or an increased period of tiredness, usually after lunch. An afternoon siesta can serve as a buffer against the post-lunch dip, revitalizing your energy levels and enhancing your overall alertness.

Nap Before a Workout or Challenging Activity

Elevate your physical and mental performance by strategically napping before engaging in a workout or confronting a challenging task. The rejuvenating effects of a nap pave the way for heightened endurance, focus, and resilience.

Avoid Napping Late in the Day

While napping holds transformative power, exercise caution when venturing into the late afternoon or early evening. Napping too close to bedtime may disrupt your nighttime sleep by reducing your adenosine levels, so it is best to avoid sleeping later in the day. Sufficient adenosine is important for getting to sleep at night and can take time to build back up, so try not to sleep too close to bedtime. If you struggle to get to sleep at night, it may be best to avoid napping altogether.

By embracing the art and science of strategic napping, you recharge your energy reserves, elevate your cognitive powers, boost your mental resilience, and maximize your waking hours.

SIX

PUTTING IT ALL TOGETHER

6.1 Recap of the 5 Steps

Embarking on the journey to transform your sleep has been a comprehensive exploration, a holistic 5-step process designed to elevate your sleep quality and overall well-being. Let's revisit each step, celebrating the essence and impact they bring to your quest for rejuvenating rest.

Step 1: Environmental Assessment

Creating a sleep-friendly environment is the cornerstone of your sleep transformation. It goes beyond aesthetics as you refine the essence of your surroundings, optimizing airflow, light exposure, and sound to eliminate sleep disturbances and sleep more efficiently. Think of it as crafting a space where every element works together to create an optimal setting for rejuvenation. By dedicating your bed solely to sleep and intimacy you set the stage for profound change.

Step 2: Schedule Alignment

Timing is crucial when it comes to sleep, and schedule alignment is the key to organising your day to facilitate better sleep. It's not just about how long you sleep; it's about aligning your daily activities with your body's natural rhythm. From consistent sleep timing to understanding Ultranean Sleep Cycles, this step empowers you to sync with the intrinsic patterns of your body, unlocking a cascade of benefits for your overall well-being.

Step 3: Tools to Get to Sleep

In a world brimming with distractions and stressors, having an arsenal of tools to guide you into the realm of sleep is invaluable. Whether it's the calming embrace of a body scan, the relaxation induced by Progressive Muscle Relaxation (PMR), or the restorative power of Non-Sleep Deep Rest (NSDR) practices, these tools are your allies. They not only facilitate the transition into sleep but also stand ready to offer solace on restless nights, ensuring you find your way back to restfulness.

Step 4: Ensuring Quality Sleep

Quality over quantity—a mantra that encapsulates the essence of Step 4. This step underscores the importance of how well you sleep. From the avoidance of heavy meals close to bedtime to steering clear of substances that can disrupt your sleep architecture, this step encourages mindful choices for a sleep experience that goes beyond the clock.

Step 5: Adjusting Sleep-Wake Times

Adjusting your sleep and waking times is a dance with your body's natural rhythms. It's not without its challenges, but the rewards are profound. From investigating potential sleep or mental health diagnoses to embracing strategic napping, this step is about aligning your internal clock with the external world and ensuring that when you sleep and wake up complements your unique Chronotype.

As we conclude this journey, remember, fixing your sleep is not a universal or standardized endeavor. It's about understanding your body, making intentional choices, and creating an environment that fosters restorative sleep. Finally, let's look into some practical aspects of implementing, maintaining, and evolving your newfound sleep strategies to achieve the ideal night's rest.

6.2 Embracing Healthier Sleep: Practical Implementation Tips

Below is a table that lists each strategy mentioned throughout this book. It is suggested that readers do not attempt to implement all strategies at once, as this will likely not be effective or sustainable. It is suggested to implement between 1-5 strategies per week, beginning with Step 1 of the book and working through each subsequent step. Remember that consistency is more important than simply trying new strategies. Strategies will be more likely to work if they are implemented consistently as it may take a few weeks before results are evident. Remember, as mentioned earlier in this book, it takes 18-21 days to begin forming a habit and 66 days to solidify it.

You may choose to highlight each strategy you plan to implement and tick them off as you work your way through the list, or write them down and put them somewhere visible in your house.

6.3 Comprehensive Sleep Strategy Toolkit Table

See below for a table summarising each sleep strategy mentioned previously in this book and whether it assists with falling asleep, staying asleep, waking up, or better sleep.

<table>
<tr><td colspan="5" align="center">Comprehensive Sleep Strategy Toolkit</td></tr>
<tr><td rowspan="2">Sleep Strategy</td><td colspan="4" align="center">What the Sleep Strategy Will Help With</td></tr>
<tr><td>Step 1: Environmental Assessment</td><td>Quality</td><td>Quantity</td><td>Regularity</td><td>Timing</td></tr>
<tr><td>Ensure Proper Ventilation</td><td>✔</td><td>✔</td><td></td><td></td></tr>
<tr><td>Dedicate your bed to sleep and intimacy</td><td>✔</td><td>✔</td><td></td><td>✔</td></tr>
<tr><td>Dim Lights below eye level at night</td><td>✔</td><td>✔</td><td>✔</td><td>✔</td></tr>
<tr><td>Blackout curtains</td><td>✔</td><td>✔</td><td>✔</td><td>✔</td></tr>
<tr><td>Avoid electronic devices within an hour of bedtime</td><td>✔</td><td></td><td></td><td>✔</td></tr>
<tr><td>Avoid clocks when trying to sleep</td><td>✔</td><td>✔</td><td></td><td></td></tr>
<tr><td>Elevate feet</td><td>✔</td><td></td><td></td><td></td></tr>
<tr><td>Sunlight exposure early in the morning</td><td>✔</td><td></td><td>✔</td><td>✔</td></tr>
<tr><td>Sunlight exposure late in the afternoon</td><td>✔</td><td></td><td>✔</td><td>✔</td></tr>
<tr><td>Avoid blue light at night</td><td>✔</td><td></td><td>✔</td><td>✔</td></tr>
<tr><td>Use an eye mask</td><td></td><td></td><td>✔</td><td>✔</td></tr>
<tr><td>Cold showers and ice baths</td><td></td><td></td><td>✔</td><td>✔</td></tr>
<tr><td>Warm showers and warm baths</td><td></td><td></td><td>✔</td><td>✔</td></tr>
<tr><td>Cool bedroom and adjustable blankets</td><td>✔</td><td>✔</td><td></td><td></td></tr>
</table>

Sleep Strategy	What the Sleep Strategy Will Help With			
Step 2: Schedule Alignment	Quality	Quantity	Regularity	Timing
Sleep a consistent number of hours each night	✔	✔	✔	
Sleep in 90-minute Ultranean Sleep Cycles	✔		✔	
Sleep to your Chronotype	✔		✔	✔
Morning cardio fitness	✔		✔	
Daytime resistance training	✔	✔		
Consistent mealtimes to match your sleep cycle	✔		✔	✔
Intermittent fasting for productivity	✔			
Avoid large meals before productive times or bedtime	✔			
Hydrate earlier in the day	✔	✔		
Develop a consistent morning routine	✔		✔	✔
Develop a consistent nighttime routine	✔	✔	✔	✔

Sleep Strategy	What the Sleep Strategy Will Help With			
Step 3: Tools to Get to Sleep	Quality	Quantity	Regularity	Timing
Body scan	✔	✔		✔
PMR protocol	✔	✔		✔
NSDR practices including naps, meditation, hypnosis and yoga nidra	✔	✔		✔
Auditory tools including nature sounds, colored noises, binaural beats, bedtime stories, ASMR and relaxing low-BPM music	✔	✔		✔
Taking a mental walk	✔	✔		✔

Sleep Strategy	What the Sleep Strategy Will Help With			
Step 4: Ensuring Quality Sleep	Quality	Quantity	Regularity	Timing
Avoid stimulating activities and engage in relaxing activities close to bedtime	✔	✔		✔
Avoid eating a small meal within 1 hour of a large meal within 2 hours of bed	✔			✔
Avoid alcohol and marijuana (particularly THC) close to sleep	✔			
Avoid caffeine within 8 to 14 hours of sleep	✔	✔		✔
Avoid caffeine within 90 minutes of waking	✔			
Avoid more than 400mg of caffeine per day	✔			
Consider abstaining from caffeine for 2-4 weeks to resensitize	✔			

Sleep Strategy	What the Sleep Strategy Will Help With			
Step 5: Adjusting Sleep-Wake Times	Quality	Quantity	Regularity	Timing
Investigate any potential sleep or mental health diagnoses	✔	✔	✔	✔
Ensure sufficient wind-down time at night	✔	✔	✔	✔
Use light exposure and cold/warm water to adjust your Circadian Rhythm	✔			✔
Identify your Chronotype and align your schedule to match it	✔	✔	✔	✔
Sleeping Backward				✔
Sleep Scheduling		✔	✔	✔
Sleeping Forward				✔
Avoid spending more than 20-25 mins lying in bed trying to sleep without a break		✔		✔
Strategic napping	✔	✔		

SEVEN
RESOURCES AND FURTHER READING

7.1 Books, Podcasts and Articles

1 Hanley, G. (Director). (21 June 2018). *Gregory Hanley, PhD, BCBA-D | Part 1 of Sleep problems of children & young adults with ASD* (Vol. 1). https://www.youtube.com/watch?v=_H1I-QEENmg

2 Hanley, G. (Director). (21 June 2018). *Gregory Hanley, PhD, BCBA-D | Part 2 of Sleep problems of children & young adults with ASD* (Vol. 2). https://www.youtube.com/watch?v=mDbb0XQDnng

3 Huberman, A. and Walker, M. (May 2024). *Guest Series special episode 1 of 6 | Dr. Matt Walker: The Biology of Sleep & Your Unique Sleep Needs.* In *Huberman Lab.* Scicomm Media. https://open.spotify.com/episode/5Afj79C1uxCrGb2MYbxsFe?si=23d8703ba3314238

4 Huberman, A. and Walker, M. (May 2024). *Guest Series special episode 2 of 6 | Dr. Matt Walker: Protocols to Improve Your Sleep.* In *Huberman Lab.* Scicomm Media. https://open.spotify.com/episode/1Ab1UcjpAvbhAhUslDt0kA?si=ceedcbd3a81a4c1d

5 Huberman, A. and Walker, M. (May 2024). *Guest Series special episode 3 of 6 | Dr. Matt Walker: How to Structure Your Sleep, Use Naps & Time Caffeine.* In *Huberman Lab.* Scicomm Media. https://open.spotify.com/episode/2mu7ZIGgdycsWpaUifPJSr?si=1ae76cf6f17d451a

6 Huberman, A. and Walker, M. (May 2024). *Guest Series special episode 4 of 6 | Dr. Matt Walker: Using Sleep to Improve Learning, Creativity & Memory.* In *Huberman Lab.* Scicomm Media. https://open.spotify.com/episode/0OzETTRh8ETwFgdKEb2lAD?si=03008b5ef5f34ae9

7 Huberman, A. and Walker, M. (May 2024). *Guest Series special episode 5 of 6 | Dr. Matt Walker: Improve Sleep and Boost Mood & Emotional Regulation.* In *Huberman Lab.* Scicomm Media. https://open.spotify.com/episode/44LuBco7xLJaPUcGDLqYfX?si=3b1720684106470b

8 Huberman, A. and Walker, M. (May 2024). *Guest Series special episode 6 of 6 | Dr. Matt Walker: The Science of Dreams and Lucid Dreaming.* In *Huberman Lab.* Scicomm Media. https://open.spotify.com/episode/02hF0APCl4oFvKITlO8fda?si=4bda5f3b5ea448c5

9 Huberman, A. (Jan 2021). *Be More Alert When Awake.* In *Huberman Lab.* Scicomm Media. https://open.spotify.com/episode/4JIM6biMG5CQDsSMQFwG3O?si=4af4012399b1450e

10 Huberman, A. (Feb 2023). *Dr. Gina Poe: Use Sleep to Enhance Learning, Memory & Emotional State.* In *Huberman Lab.* Scicomm Media. https://open.spotify.com/episode/3RWeArnFqgOOE62oJnDt0r?si=BaOk7EHDSKOjPvfGTUHFkw

11 Huberman, A. (Aug 2021). *Dr. Matthew Walker: The Science & Practice of Perfecting Your Sleep.* In *Huberman Lab.* Scicomm Media. https://open.spotify.com/episode/

4KNsmuCgX6lz8GE2J3393Y?si=
Mk2N51eVRJqAHr0B2qv3Sw

12 Huberman, A. (Jan 2021). *How to Defeat Jetlag, Shift Work & Sleeplessness*. In *Huberman Lab*. Scicomm Media. https://open.spotify.com/episode/5M2X4GKJEqi2Fgj8NBz4yG?si=ebf71fd084aa44a6

13 Huberman, A. (Aug 2022). *Sleep Toolkit: Tools for Optimizing Sleep & Sleep-Wake Timing*. In *Huberman Lab*. Scicomm Media. https://open.spotify.com/episode/3TxjF2mZy9S9I9GL5eZ8sq?si=IqTsxDKWSk-QOa06OCC5hA

14 Huberman, A. (Feb 2021). *Understanding and Using Dreams to Learn and to Forget*. In *Huberman Lab*. Scicomm Media. https://open.spotify.com/episode/61Lak7dzmChM8sc5mkr0yZ?si=b438a498d2c84683

15 Huberman, A. (Jan 2021). *Using Science to Optimize Learning, Sleep & Metabolism*. In *Huberman Lab*. Scicomm Media. https://open.spotify.com/episode/3eV2VGviKclKdRymfYS8Ae?si=7debe1d09aa349c6

16 Kaskie, R. E., Graziano, B., & Ferrarelli, F. (2017). Schizophrenia and sleep disorders: Links, risks and management challenges. *Nature and Science of Sleep*, *9*, 227–239.

17 Lin, Y. S., Weibel, J., Landolt, H. P., Santini, F., Garbazza, C., Kistler, J., Rehm, S., Rentsch, K., Borgwardt, S., Cajochen, C & Reichert, C. F. (2022). Time to recover from daily caffeine intake. *Frontiers in Nutrition*, 8 (787225), 1-11.

18 Roehrs, T., & Roth, T. (2008). Caffeine: sleep and daytime sleepiness. *Sleep medicine reviews*, 12(2), 153-162.

19 Shanahan, P., Palod, S., Smith, K., Fife-Schaw, C., & Mirza, N. (2019). Interventions for sleep difficulties in adults with an intellectual disability: A systematic review. *Journal of Intellectual Disability Research*, *63*(5), 372–385.

20 Waite, F., Myers, E., Harvey, A. G., Espie, C. A., Startup, H., Sheaves, B., & Freeman, D. (2016). Treating sleep problems in Schizophrenia. *Behavioural and Cognitive Psychotherapy*, *44*(3), 273–287.

21 Walker, M. (2018). *Why we sleep*. Penguin Books.

22 Weibel, J., Lin, Y. S., Landolt, H. P., Kistler, J., Rehm, S., Rentsch, K. M., Slawik, H., Borgwardt, S., Cajochen, C. and Reichert, C. F. (2021). The impact of daily caffeine intake on nighttime sleep in young adult men. *Scientific reports*, 11(4668), 1-9.

23 Wiggs, L., & France, K. (2000). Behavioural treatments for sleep problems in children and adolescents with physical illness, psychological problems or intellectual disabilities. *Sleep Medicine Reviews*, *4*(3), 299–314.

7.2 Apps and Tools for Better Sleep

Insight Timer for guided meditation - https://insighttimer.com/

Headspace for guided meditation - https://www.headspace.com/headspace-meditation-app

Yoga Nidra Script 1 - https://www.youtube.com/watch?v=M0u9GST_j3s&t=48s

Yoga Nidra Script 2 - https://www.youtube.com/watch?v=FroVfmOtaps

Reveri for Clinically Backed Hypnosis Scripts - https://
www.reveri.com/

Morningness-Eveningness Questionnaire (MEQ) - https://
qxmd.com/calculate/calculator_829/morningness-
eveningness-questionnaire-meq

Try out the Rise app to help you get your sleep on track -
https://www.risescience.com/

ABOUT THE AUTHOR

Edwin Gall is an experienced behavior specialist, with a social science degree and a passion for helping others. He has dedicated many years to understanding the complexities of human behavior and the mind. Drawing from his extensive background, Edwin now leverages his expertise to empower individuals to overcome obstacles, achieve personal growth, and optimize their overall well-being as a life coach. With a compassionate approach rooted in years of hands-on experience, Edwin is committed to guiding others toward a life of fulfillment and success. His background uniquely positions him to offer invaluable insights and strategies for managing sleep challenges and optimizing overall well-being.